Dr. Mom's

Essential Oils
First Aid

COPING WITH NON-EMERGENCY MISHAPS IN A NATURAL WAY!

Judy Jehn, RMT & Brenda Sheldon, RMT

Vision Publishing, LLC
Denver, CO

Copyright © 2011 by Judy Jehn

2nd Edition, August, 2011

Kathryn Caywood, LLC, Editor

Ann Zielinski, Book Design

International Standard Book Number: ISBN 978-0-9818290-1-2

Library of Congress Control Number: 2011934573

Jehn, Judy

Dr. Mom's Essential Oils First Aid / Judy Jehn, Brenda Sheldon

1. Essential Oils. 2. Aromatherapy. 3. First Aid.

Printed in USA

VisionPublishingLLC.com

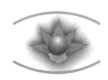

Contents

Nature's Original Medicine

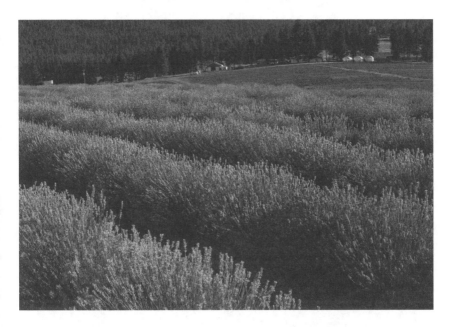

Essential Oils

What are Essential Oils?

- Aromatic liquids of plants, trees, leaves, fruit, and flowers

- Natural oils that have nutritional and therapeutic properties

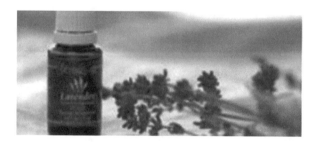

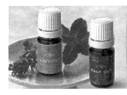 

- Essential Oils have the ability to

  - Prevent and relieve the discomforts associated with a wide variety of health problems

  - Reduce stress

  - Lift depression and restore or enhance a sense of well-being

  - Provide revitalizing beauty-care treatments for skin, hair, and body

Phyto = Plant

- **Phytochemical** - the plant's active chemical components (constituents) that account for its medicinal properties
  - Mosby's Medical Dictionary, 8th edition. © 2009, Elsevier.

- **Phytonutrient** and phytochemical are used interchangeably to describe those plant compounds which are thought to have health-enhancing qualities

- More terms: **Phytomedicinal** and **phytotherapy**

Essential Oils
Have the Ability to Influence

Phyto-nutritionally

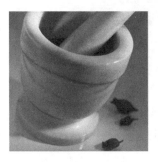

Physiologically

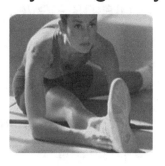

Psychologically

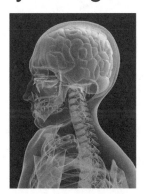

Phyto-nutritionally

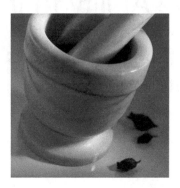

- The human body is made up of proteins - every cell from toenails to hair

- Essential oils are compounds containing amino acids which convert to protein

- When cells are compromised, essential oils start regeneration through the healing properties of amino acids and the increased oxygen to the tissues

Physiologically

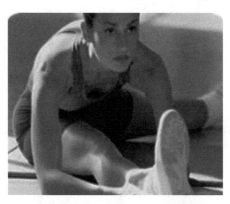

- Essential oils support different areas of the body, for example:
  - Numerous oils from herbs assist in strengthening and realignment of the musculoskeletal system
  - Various oils from spices benefit the digestive and immune systems
  - Many oils can break down and detoxify the chemical build up in fatty tissue, potentially clearing DNA

Essential Oils Promote Homeostasis

Psychologically

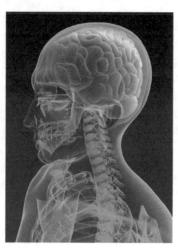

- Through the sense of smell, essential oils soothe the mind and calm the psyche, producing a restorative effect on the emotions

- Some essential oils stimulate the neurotransmitters of the brain

Quality Makes the Difference

- "100% Pure" doesn't mean the same thing in the cosmetic industry

- In the U.S. only 5% real oil needs to be present to be labeled "100% Pure"

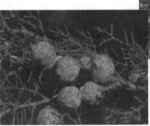

Creating a Quality Essential Oil: Every essential oil is made up of compounds (also called constituents) that are unique to that oil; and those constituents are what make the oil therapeutic grade. For example, cypress oil has 280 known constituents. If the oil is distilled for 20 hours, only 20 of the properties are present. If the oil is distilled for 26 hours, zero properties appear. Correctly distilling cypress for 24 hours allows all of the 280 constituents to be present.

Fingerprinting Methods

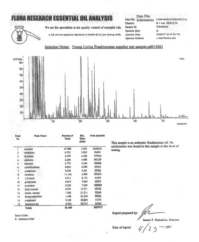 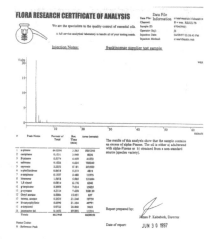

Testing for Purity

- Gas chromatography
- Mass spectroscopy
- Thin layer chromatography
- High performance liquid chromatography

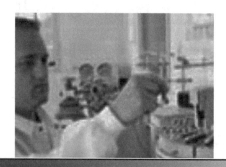

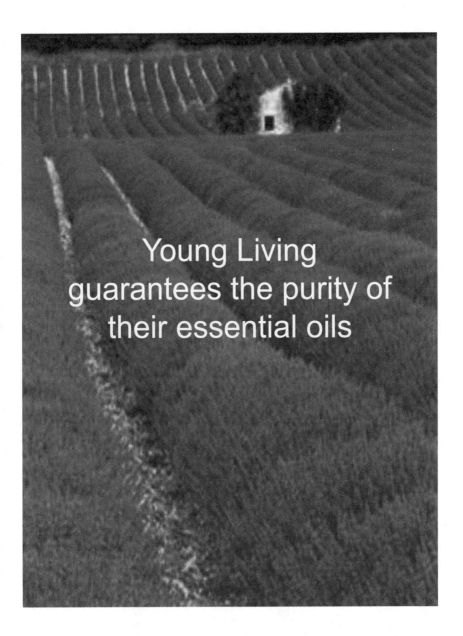

Young Living guarantees the purity of their essential oils

Dr. Mom

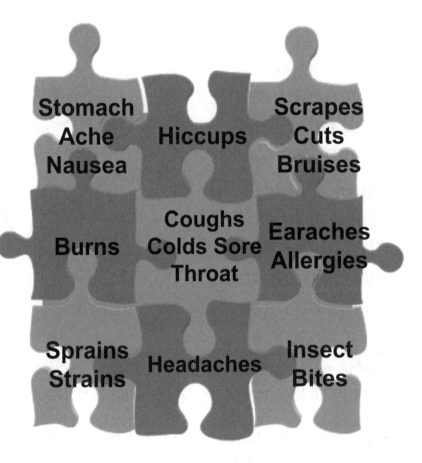

Stomach Ache Nausea

Hiccups

Scrapes Cuts Bruises

Burns

Coughs Colds Sore Throat

Earaches Allergies

Sprains Strains

Headaches

Insect Bites

Technique

Allergies

- Combine lavender and Roman chamomile 50:50

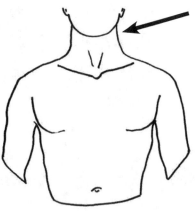

- Apply two or three drops of this blend on the wrists or on the sides of the throat (carotid artery)

Hint: In an empty 5ml bottle, mix 20 drops of each oil, then fill the rest of the bottle with V-6 Mixing Oil
- Use on the bottoms of the feet for a relaxing foot massage for restless legs
- Place one or two drops on a cotton ball or on the sheet in a baby's crib or bassinet to calm a stressful baby

---

Technique

Bruises

- For bruising (or possibility of bruising), use 1 or 2 drops of one of the following oils
  - Geranium
  - Helichrysum
  - Lavender

- Gently rub into tissue, across the bruise first in one direction several times, and then in the other direction

- Apply Regenolone and gently flush up towards the heart

To prevent bruising, apply as soon as possible after injury

Technique

Minor Burns and Sunburn

- For 1st and 2nd degree burns

  - Lavender, lavender, lavender!

  - Other oils: Idaho balsam fir, helichrysum, and Believe reduce scarring and tissue discoloration and support tissue regeneration

  - KidScents Lotion, LavaDerm Cooling Mist Spray, Liquid Stevia, and Mineral Essence assist in the healing process

Caution: For 3rd degree burns (and/ or shock), seek immediate medical attention!

Is it a Cold or the Flu?

- Common cold, including chest cold and head cold, can be caused by one of more than 200 viruses

- Seasonal flu can be caused by either influenza A or B viruses

- The common cold and flu are both contagious viral infections of the respiratory tract

It's a virus!

Source: WebMD

Cold Viruses

- Rhinoviruses - the worst offenders

- Most active in early fall, spring, and summer

- More than 110 distinct rhinovirus types

- Grow best at temperatures of about 91 degrees, that perfect body temperature right inside the human nose

- Seldom produce serious illnesses

Other cold viruses, such as parainfluenza, produce mild infections in adults but can lead to severe lower respiratory infections, such as pneumonia, in young children

Source: WebMD

Cold Viruses

- Coronaviruses, another cold producing virus, cause a large percentage of adult colds

  - Most active in the winter and early spring

  - Unlike rhinoviruses, they are difficult to grow in the laboratory

- The causes of 30% to 50% of adult colds, presumed to be viral, remain unidentified

Source: WebMD

Cold Viruses

- There is no evidence that you can get a cold from

  - Exposure to cold weather or from getting chilled or overheated

  - Related factors such as exercise, diet, or enlarged tonsils or adenoids

- Research suggests that

  - Psychological stress and allergic diseases affecting your nose or throat may have an impact on your chances of getting infected by cold viruses

Source: WebMD

Flu Viruses

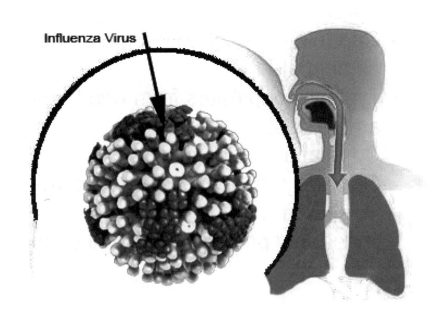

Influenza enters through the nose and settles in the respiratory tract.

Flu Viruses

- Type A flu or influenza A viruses

  - Capable of infecting people as well as animals
  - Typically originates from wild birds as the hosts
  - Constantly changing
  - Generally responsible for the large flu epidemics
  - Spread by people who are already infected

Type B flu is found only in humans
  - Type B flu may cause a less severe reaction than type A flu virus
  - Occasionally, type B flu can still be extremely harmful
  - Influenza type B viruses are not classified by subtype and do not cause pandemics

Source: WebMD

Cold vs. Flu

- Since both diseases are viral, antibiotics cannot conquer cold or flu

- A few antiviral medications are available to treat flu

- There are no medications that specifically defeat the common cold

- Antibiotics may be helpful only if there is a secondary bacterial infection

Although the symptoms can be similar, flu is much worse. A cold may drag you down a bit, but the flu can make you shudder at the very thought of getting out of bed.

Source: WebMD

What is the solution?

Prevention
with
Essential Oils!

Coughs, Colds, and Congestion

- Estimates are that we come in contact with 100 different cold germs daily

- The average child suffers from 6 - 10 colds per year

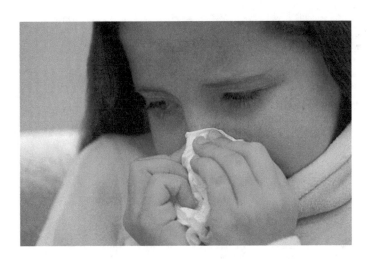

Technique

Coughs, Colds, and Congestion

- Diffuse, Diffuse, Diffuse!

  - Thieves, R.C., Purification, Raven, *Eucalyptus radiata*, frankincense, *Melaleuca alternifolia* (tea tree), lavender, Melrose

  - Lemon with cedarwood

  - Lemon with myrtle

  - Lemon with copaiba

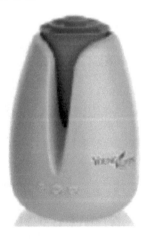

  - Myrtle with copaiba

Source: Essential Oils Desk Reference

Technique

Coughs, Colds, and Congestion

- Thieves on the feet!

- Dilute with carrier oil, like V-6, and apply to throat and chest: *Eucalyptus globulus* (do not use on infants or young children), frankincense, ginger, lemon, myrrh, peppermint (be sure to dilute well for children's sensitive skin), rosemary, sandalwood, Thieves, or Melrose

- On the spine, use Raven, or layer lemon and thyme; feather up the spine "Raindrop" style; cover immediately with OrthoEase Massage Oil or V-6 Mixing Oil

Source: Essential Oils Desk Reference

Technique

Sore Throat

- *Melaleuca alternifolia* (tea tree), copaiba, Raven, Thieves, cypress, *Eucalyptus radiata*, lemon, frankincense, thyme, oregano, peppermint, myrrh, wintergreen, Melrose

- Diffuse 2 - 3 times daily

- Inhale 2 - 3 times daily

- Ingest in a spoonful of agave or honey

- Gargle with Thieves Mouthwash 4-8 times a day

Source: Essential Oils Desk Reference

Sore Throat "Shooters"

- Fill 5/8 dram (2 ml sample bottle) with Melrose

- Hold the bottle between thumb and middle finger, tap bottom of bottle to "shoot" the oil into the back of the throat

- Roll the back of your tongue around to help spread the oil, coating your throat

- Repeat every 10 minutes for 2 hours

- Continue as necessary

Source: Dr. Daniel Pénoël

Technique

Cuts, Scrapes and Abrasions

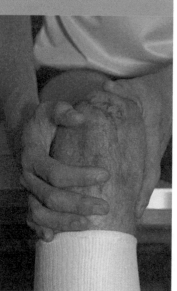

- Use helichrysum or dorado azul to stop the bleeding

- Cleansing the wound
  - Mix Thieves Household Cleaner with water, ratio 1 to 30, in a spray bottle
  - OR, fill an empty Thieves Spray bottle with
    - ½ oz Thieves Fresh Essence Plus Mouthwash
    - ½ oz distilled water

See the Essential Oils Desk Reference for more ideas

30

Technique

Cuts, Scrapes and Abrasions

- To support wound healing, fill an 8 oz spray bottle with distilled water, add

  - ¼ tsp Thieves Household Cleaner

  - 4-6 drops Purification, *Melaleuca alternifolia* (tea tree), or Melrose

DO NOT USE *Melaleuca alternifolia* (tea tree) or Melrose on puncture wounds—use clove, Thieves, rosemary, or cistus

Technique

Cuts, Scrapes and Abrasions

- SCAR-B-GONE Recipe
  - 10 drops helichrysum
  - 6 drops lavender
  - 8 drops lemongrass
  - 4 drops patchouli
  - 5 drops myrrh
  - 1 oz V-6 Enhanced Vegetable Oil Complex

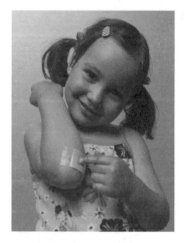

Courtesy of Nancy Sanderson

Earaches

- Otitis media (ear infection) - inflammation of middle ear from fluid build up

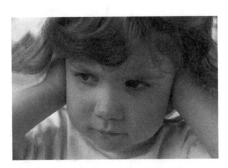

- Causes – germs from colds, sore throats, or other respiratory problems

- Can be bacterial or viral, intensely painful

- In the US, 93% of all children have had at least one acute episode by age 7, 50% of children by age 1

- Cost - $3 billion a year because of increasing resistance to antibiotics

Earaches

- Possible triggers

  - Exposure to tobacco smoke; second-hand smoke causes 22 - 27% of all cases

  - Household mold

  - Food allergies

  - Dairy products

Technique

Earaches

- Dilute 50-50 lemon, Exodus II, or Raven, rub gently around the *outside* of the ear and over the lymph nodes on the side of the neck

- Lavender, *Melaleuca alternifolia* (tea tree), chamomile, Purification, or Melrose - put a few drops of oil onto a cotton ball, gently place in the ear, and replace with a fresh cotton ball 2 - 3 times per day until the infection is gone

Caution: Never place oils directly in the ears

Technique

Earaches

- More essential oil blends to consider to calm a stressed-out child in pain:

  - Blends:
    - Peace & Calming
    - Gentle Baby

  - Roll-ons:
    - Stress Away
    - Tranquil

- For infants and small children, apply to your hands and over your heart, or along your neck, then hold and comfort the child while caressing

Headache

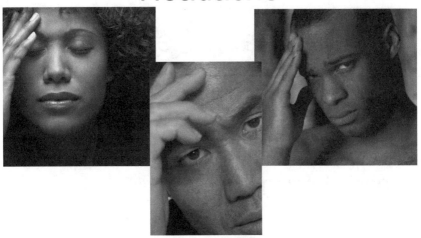

- Acetaminophen overdose is the leading cause of liver failure in the US and the UK

- Studies indicate that acetaminophen overdose results in over 56,000 injuries, 2,500 hospitalizations, and an estimated 450 deaths per year

- Overdose may overwhelm the liver's defenses and cause liver damage or even liver failure

- The only known cure for acute liver failure is a liver transplant

Technique

Simple Headache Solutions

- Use your favorite roll-on along the occipital ridge

  - Breathe Again

  - Deep Relief

  - RutaVaLa

  - Stress Away

  - Tranquil

  - Valor

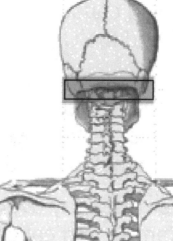

Technique

Simple Headache Solutions

- Peppermint, peppermint, peppermint!

- Wintergreen, Pan Away, M-Grain

- Other oils:
    - Roman chamomile

    - lavender

    - spearmint

    - valerian

    - clove

    - rosemary

Technique

Reflexology
Points for Headache

Apply essential oil and gently hold or
rub for 30 - 60 seconds

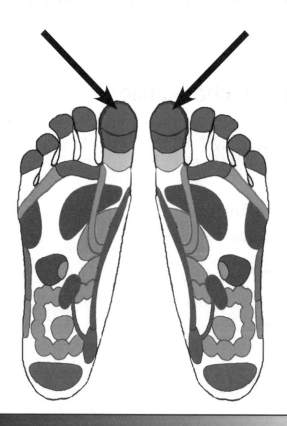

Reflexology
Points for Headache

Apply essential oil and gently press
thumbs together for 30 - 60 seconds

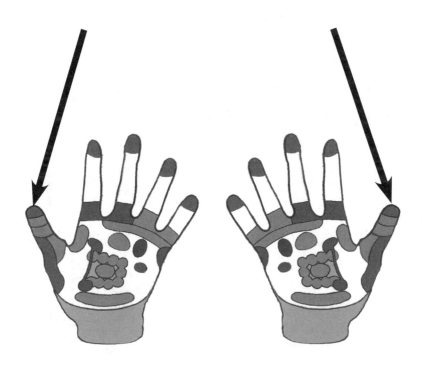

Technique

Acupressure Points for Headache

- Apply essential oils to the "web" area between thumb and finger

- With thumb and finger from opposite hand, find the "tender" spot

- Hold gently for 30 - 60 seconds or longer if necessary

Hint: This technique works best when someone else does it to you! Ask them to do both hands!

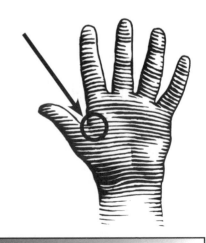

Vascular or Migraine Headaches

- **Vascular or migraine** - the vast majority may be due to colon congestion or poor digestion
  - M-Grain
  - wintergreen
  - helichrysum
  - rosemary
  - peppermint
  - lavender
  - marjoram
  - Eucaluptus globulus
  - PanAway
  - Clarity

- For **eyestrain and decreased vision,** try dried wolfberries because they contain large amounts of lutein, which is vital for healthy vision

Source: Essential Oils Desk Reference

Sinus Headaches

- Single oils:
  - *Eucalyptus radiata*
  - peppermint
  - rosemary
  - tea tree (*Melaleuca alternifolia*)
  - lavender
  - geranium

- Blends:
  - R.C.
  - Raven

- Roll-ons:
  - Breathe Again
  - Tranquil
  - Deep Relief

Technique

"Raccoon Mask"
Sinus Headache or Infection

- Use 2 - 3 drops of oil in the palm of your hand
- With pinky finger, dot around eyes and under nose
- Rub palms together, cup hands over nose, inhale, relax

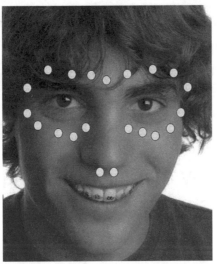

Caution: Keep oils about an inch away from the eyes

Technique

Nasal Irrigation Regimen for Sinus Headache or Infection

- Use rosemary and tea tree (*Melaleuca alternifolia*) in a saline solution
    - 10 drops rosemary
    - 6 drops tea tree (*Melaleuca alternifolia*)
    - 8 Tbs very fine salt (sometimes called salt flower)

- Thoroughly mix oils with salt, keep in a tightly sealed glass container

Source: Essential Oils Desk Reference

Technique

Nasal Irrigation Regimen for Sinus Headache or Infection

- For each nasal irrigation session, dissolve 1 tsp of salt mixture into 1 ½ C distilled water

- Use a Neti Pot or nasal irrigator to irrigate nasal cavities (follow the instructions of the manufacturer)

> Another option is to use a nasal sprayer

Source: Essential Oils Desk Reference

Tension Headaches

- Single Oils:
    - lavender
    - Roman chamomile
    - valerian
    - tangerine
    - jasmine
    - geranium
    - frankincense
    - peppermint

- Blends:
    - Aroma Siez
    - M-Grain
    - Peace & Calming
    - Hope
    - Sacred Mountain
    - Trauma Life
    - Relieve It
    - Clarity
    - PanAway

- Roll-ons:
    - Stress Away
    - Tranquil
    - Deep Relief
    - RutaVaLa
    - Valor

Source: Essential Oils Desk Reference

Technique

Tension Headaches

- Massage essential oil (dilute with carrier oil as necessary) along the back of the neck, base of the skull, down the sides of the neck, and onto the shoulders
- Apply to temples and across forehead
- Rub hands together and run fingers through hair from behind the ears to the top of the skull

- Massage whole skull, especially where it hurts

- Cup hands over nose and mouth and breathe deeply

- Lie down for a few minutes and think, "My head is feeling better!"

Headache Notes

Technique

Hiccups

- Place tarragon, cypress, or spearmint on the esophagus in the clavicle notch (A)

- Blend 50-50 lavender and Roman chamomile; place on the diaphragm just below the sternum (B), using four fingers on each hand in an upside down "V shape," curve fingers around the ribs and hold

Technique

Insect Bites and Stings

"Bugging" bugs with non-toxic repellents!

- Peppermint
- Cedarwood
- Lemongrass
- Geranium
- Lavender
- Pine
- Cinnamon

- Rosemary
- Thyme
- Palo santo
- Idaho tansy

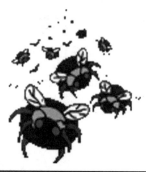

Technique

Insect Bites and Stings

- Bees, wasps, hornets - Purification, Thieves, PanAway, Idaho tansy, Melrose, *Melaleuca alternifolia* (tea tree)

- Ticks - Purification, lemongrass

- Flies - Rosemary, peppermint (repellent)

- Mosquitoes - Lavender, lemongrass, peppermint

- Brown Recluse Spider - Helichrysum, Thieves

Technique

Nausea

- Patchouli contains compounds that are effective in preventing vomiting because of their ability to reduce gastrointestinal muscle contractions

- Other oils:
    - peppermint
    - ginger
    - wintergreen
    - Idaho tansy
    - Di-Gize

Source: Essential Oils Desk Reference

Technique

Nausea

- Mild nausea can be relieved by applying acupressure on the inside of your wrist

- Place your thumb three fingers up from the bend in your wrist, between the two tendons

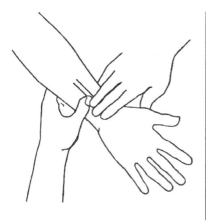

Put a little patchouli or peppermint on the area before applying the acupressure

Technique

Sprains and Strains

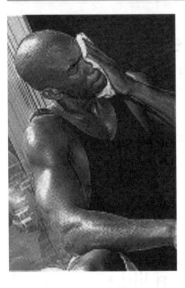

- PanAway!

- Layer peppermint, Believe, and geranium every 10 – 15 minutes for the first few hours; then, 3- 5 times per day

- Other oils: copaiba, marjoram, lavender, wintergreen, Roman chamomile, Aroma Siez, Aroma Life

- Roll-ons: Deep Relief, Stress Away

Technique

More Help
for
Sprains and Strains

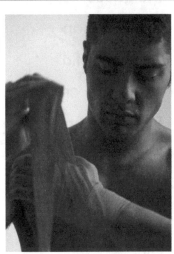

- OrthoEase Massage Oil and OrthoSport Massage Oil
  - Anti-inflammatory and pain-killing complex
  - Ideal for strained, swollen, or torn muscles and ligaments

- Regenolone Moisturizing Creamprovides relief from all types of arthritis, muscle and skeletal pain

For more information on sprains and strains, see the *Weekend Warrior-Winning With Essential Oils* CD or the Essential Oils Companion booklet.

Stomach Ache
Various Causes

- Indigestion
- Constipation
- Stomach "flu"
- Menstrual cramps
- Food poisoning
- Food allergies
- Gas
- Lactose intolerance
- Ulcers
- Pelvic inflammatory disease

- Hernia
- Gallstones
- Kidney stones
- Endometriosis
- Crohn's disease
- Urinary tract infection
- Gastroesophgeal reflux disease (GERD)
- Appendicitis

Caution: If pain or discomfort persists, consult a health care practitioner

Technique

Simple Stomache Ache Solutions

- Single Oils:
  - peppermint
  - fennel
  - thyme

- Blends:
  - Di-Gize

- Apply 3 to 10 drops to abdominal area and around navel,
  dilute with carrier oil as needed,
  do light abdominal massage

- Other:
  - Digest + Cleanse soft gels
  - Longevity soft gels

Source: Essential Oils Desk Reference

Technique

Stomache Ache
Light Abdominal
Massage Technique

Use the "I L U" technique (hint: look at the diagrams upside-down!)

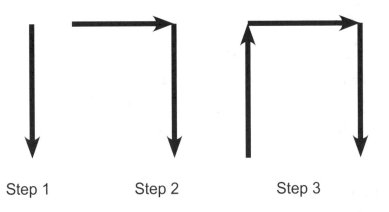

Step 1   Step 2   Step 3

Caution: If pain or discomfort increases, stop immediately and consult a health care practitioner

Technique

Stomache Ache
Light Abdominal
Massage Technique

- It's like squeezing the contents out of a sausage, you would start at the end squeezing out the contents and continuously move backwards to squeeze out the next section

- With this massage technique, do not use extreme pressure; gentle is the rule

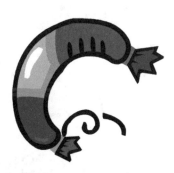

Technique

Stomache Ache Light Abdominal Massage Technique

- On the person's left side, <u>gently</u> massage DOWN the descending colon

- Start at the arrowhead and massage downward

- Move your hands <u>up</u> a "segment" and massage downward out to the end

- Continue the "segments" until you have covered this side

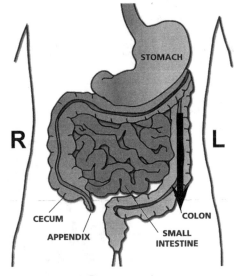

Step 1

Technique

Stomache Ache
Light Abdominal
Massage Technique

- Use the same "segment" procedure for ACROSS the transverse colon and continue DOWN the descending colon

- Start at the step 2 arrow tip on the person's left side, massage the arrow tip and DOWN the left side

- Back up a "segment" on the step 2 arrow, massage ACROSS and continue DOWN the descending colon

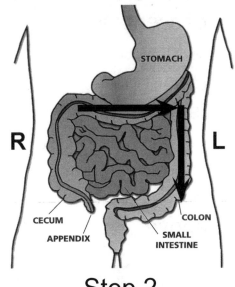

Step 2

Technique

Stomache Ache
Light Abdominal
Massage Technique

- Use the same "segment" procedure as before for UP the ascending colon on the person's right side

- Start with the step 3 arrow tip, massage UP, then ACROSS from the person's right to left along the transverse colon, and DOWN the descending colon

- Back up a "segment" on the step 3 arrow and continue as above

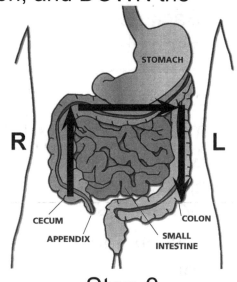

Step 3

Toothaches

- Clove, Roman chamomile, wintergreen, Melrose, PanAway, Stress Away roll-on

- Thieves or Fresh Essence mouthwash on a cotton ball between cheek and gum

- Thieves toothpaste - Dentarome, Dentarome Plus, Dentarome Ultra, KidScents Toothpaste

Items to Add to Your First Aid Kit

- Everyday Oils Collection
  - Lavender, peppermint, lemon, frankincense, Thieves, Valor, PanAway, Peace & Calming, and Purification

- Golden Touch I Kit
  - Di-Gize, Endoflex, Juvaflex, Thieves, Melrose, R.C., Raven

For home or on the road

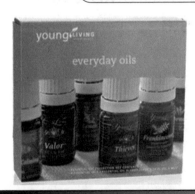
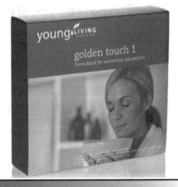

More Ideas for Your First Aid Kit

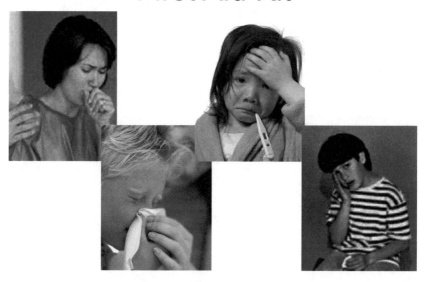

- Helichrysum or dorado azul
- Believe
- LavaDerm
- Geranium
- Clove
- Copaiba
- Deep Relief Roll-on
- Stress Away Roll-on

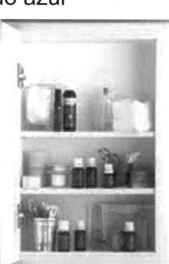

Creating a Healthier Environment for Your Family

Creating a Toxic-Free Household

- Stop eating pesticide-ridden fruits and vegetables

- Avoid over-the-counter health care products containing synthetic ingredients that are poisoning your family

Pesticides on Popular Produce

(in order of pesticide toxicity 100=highest pesticide load)

- Peaches - 100
- Strawberries - 89
- Apples - 88
- Spinach - 85
- Nectarines - 85
- Celery - 83
- Pears - 80
- Cherries - 76
- Potatoes - 67
- Sweet Bell Peppers - 66
- Raspberries - 66
- Grapes - Imported from outside U.S. - 64
- Carrots - 57
- Green Beans - 57
- Hot Peppers - 55
- Oranges - 53
- Apricots - 51
- Cucumbers - 51
- Tomatoes - 48
- Collard Greens - 48

More information …
http://www.foodnews.org/fulllist.php

Why Should We Change Our Personal Care Products?

- "If you can't eat it, don't wear it, and don't put it on your skin"*

- Everything you put in your mouth or on your head and skin goes directly into your blood stream

> Please carefully read the labels on your personal care products. If you cannot pronounce it, it probably is not good for you!

*Source: D. Gary Young

Sodium Lauryl Sulfate

- In most toothpaste, shampoo, bubble bath, liquid soaps, and detergents
- Skin irritant - A single drop can be retained in tissues up to <u>five days</u>
- Causes improper eye development in children - Dr. Keith Green
- Can react with other ingredients to form NDELA, a nitrosamine and potent carcinogen
- Researchers estimate the nitrate absorption of one shampoo is equal to eating a pound of bacon!
- FDA warning about unacceptable levels of dioxin in shampoos containing SLS
- Can enhance the allergic response to other toxins and allergens
  - Dangerous Beauty by David Lowell Kern

Propylene Glycol

- Used in cosmetics as a humectant - it helps to retain moisture

- Is "industrial antifreeze" and the major ingredient in brake and hydraulic fluid

- Known strong skin irritant

- Warning in Material Safety Data Sheets (MSDS) - absorption through skin contact can cause liver abnormalities and kidney damage

> For more information on the Dirty Dozen toxic chemicals in consumer products, go to: http://www.preventcancer.com/consumers/general/dirty_dozen.htm or refer to the brochure *Toxin Awareness* available from Sound Concepts

What's in Your Baby's Diaper Cream?

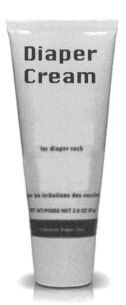

Ingredients:
Water, Mineral Oil, Dimethicone, Glycerin, Lanolin, Petrolatum, Sorbitan Isostearate, Panthenol, Oat Kernel Flour (*Avena sativa*), Microcrystalline Wax, Synthetic Beeswax, Tocopheryl Acetate, Sodium Lactate, Magnesium Sulfate, Lactic Acid, DMDM Hydantoin, Iodopropynyl Butylcarbamate

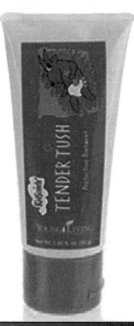

Tender Tush Ingredients:
Coconut oil, cocoa butter, beeswax, wheat germ oil, olive oil, almond oil, and the pure therapeutic grade essential oils of sandalwood, rosewood, Roman chamomile, lavender, cistus, blue tansy, and frankincense

What's Best for Your Kids?

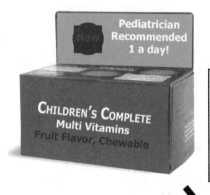

Ingredients Include:
Red Dye #40
Yellow Dye #6
Blue Dye #2
Aluminum
Aspartame

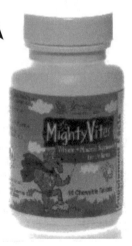

MightyVites:
Whole food, multi-nutrient that contains
super fruits, plants, and vegetables
that deliver the full spectrum of
vitamins, minerals, antioxidants, and
phytonutrients

What is in Your Baby's and Children's Shampoo?

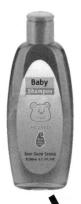

Ingredients:
  Water, PEG-80 Sorbitan Laurate, Cocamidopropyl Betaine, Sodium Trideceth Sulfate, Glycerin, Lauroamphoglycinate, PEG-150 Distearate, Sodium Laureth-13 Carboxylate, Fragrance, Polyquaternium-10, Tetrasodium EDTA, Quaternium-15, Citric Acid, D&C Yellow #10, D&C Orange #4

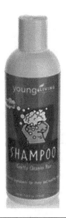

KidScents Shampoo ingredients include:
Aloe, MSM, botanical extracts, essential oils

Which Pain Relieving Products?

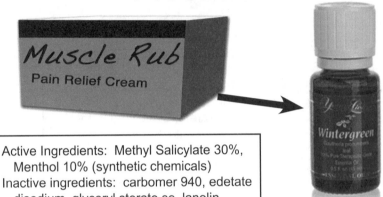

Active Ingredients: Methyl Salicylate 30%, Menthol 10% (synthetic chemicals)
Inactive ingredients: carbomer 940, edetate disodium, glyceryl sterate se, lanolin, polysorbate 80, potassium hydroxide, purified water, stearic acid, and trolamine

Natural Methyl Salicylate: 90+%

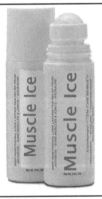

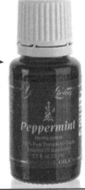

Active Ingredients:
  Natural Menthol 3.5%
Inactive Ingredients: Carbomer, FD and C blue#1, yellow #5, glycerin, herbal extract, isopropyl alcohol USP, methlparaben, natural camphor USPP, propylene glycol, silicon dioxide, triethnolamine, water

Natural Menthol: 34-44%

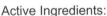

Why Over-medicate?

Studies indicate the treatment was either no better than the placebo or caused other discomforting side-effects

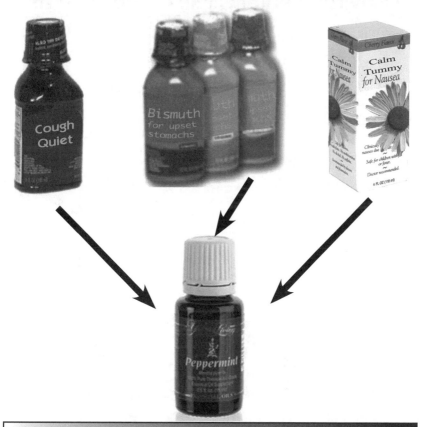

What's Under Your Sink?

- Bleach is the biggest asthmatic trigger and harmful to children, even on their toys

- The Center for Disease Control and the Association of Occupational and Environmental Clinics list bleach as one of the chemical disinfectants that cause RADS - Reactive Airways Dysfunction Syndrome or Occupational Asthma

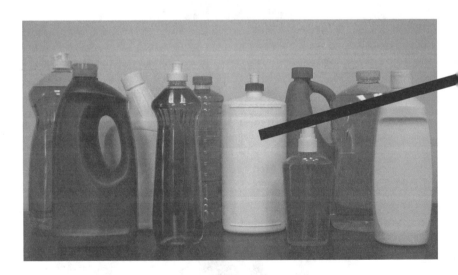

What's Under Your Sink?

Household cleaners fall under the Hazardous Products Act from the mid-1960s, which places the responsibility on the manufacturer!

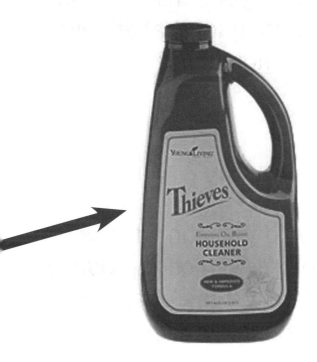

Safe, effective, germ-killing, very economical, and smells good!

Question?

What quality athletic equipment do you buy for your children if they are competing for that athletic scholarship?

Why?

What should you consider when buying your health care products for your family if the goal is long distance health?

How Do I Afford It?

Use your present budget

Each month begin to transfer a few products at a time to quality products that are health enhancing

Same budget - better choices!

How Much is Your Family's Health Worth?

Remember...
there is a difference

Young Living is an excellent choice to consider

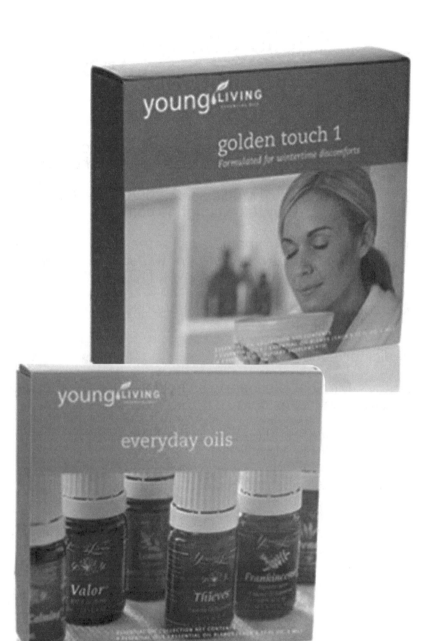

Bibliography and Webliography

Essential Oils Desk Reference, 5th ed., Life Science Publishing, 2011, www.LifeSciencePublishers.com

Gale Encyclopedia of Medicine. © 2008, The Gale Group, Inc., www.gale.cengage.com

Jehn, Judy, RMT. *Aromatherapy for the Soul—Spiritual and Emotional Empowerment with Essential Oils,* Vision Publishing, LLC, Denver, CO, 2008

McDanel, Connie and Michael, various presentations and newsletters

MedicineNet.com, 1999

Mosby's Medical Dictionary, 8th edition. © 2009, Elsevier, www.medterms.com

Stewart, David. Healing Oils of the Bible, CARE Publications, Marble Hill, MO, 2003

Young, D. Gary. Essential Oils Integrative Medical Guide, Essential Science Publishing, USA, 2003

Young, D. Gary. Aromatherapy: The Essential Beginning, 2nd ed. Essential Science Publishing, Orem, UT, 1996

General Index

Technique Index

Notes

Notes